Renal Diet Soup&Salad

A Kidney Patient's Guide to Eating Delicious, Simple, and Healthy Meals

LAUREL LAMBERT

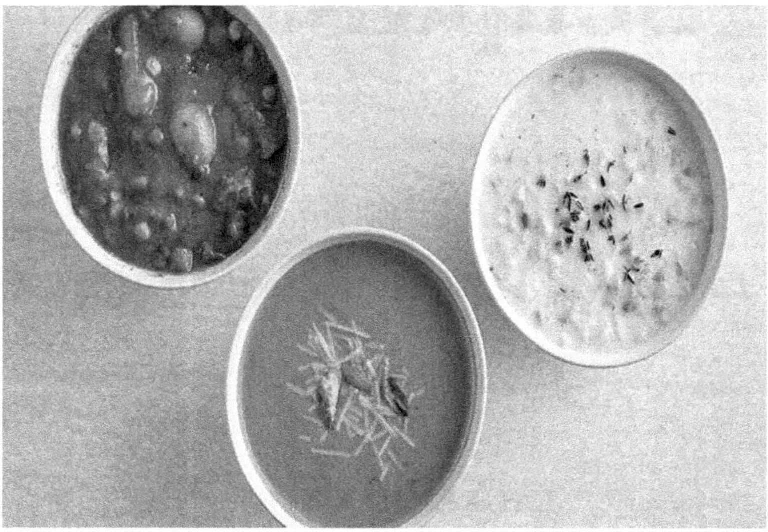

About the Author:

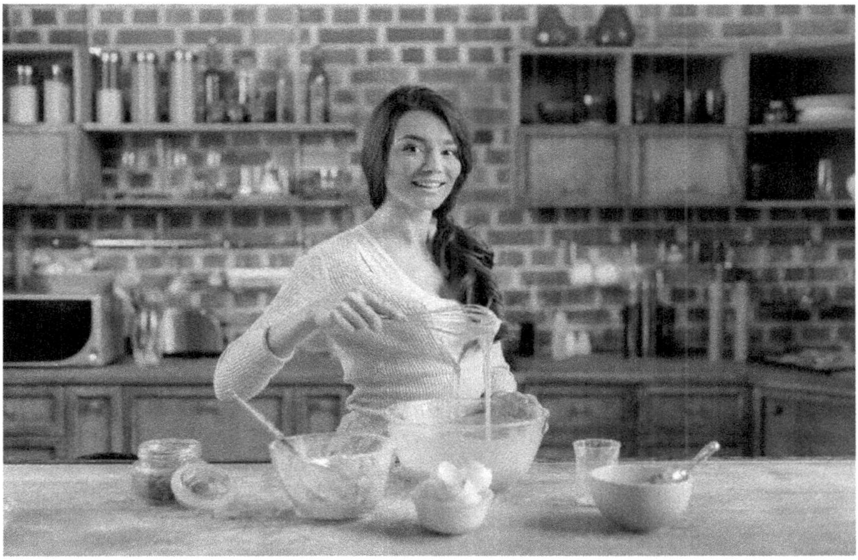

Laurel is a **nutrition expert** and a bestselling author of cookbooks, including a set of renal diet cookbooks that help people **with renal disorder** meet the food and fluid recommendations set by their doctors and dietitians:

She is an **American bestselling** cookbook author, food writer, cook, and food equity advocate. She lectures on food and residential cooking and has contributed to several others together or as a writer about health culture and mental health

Once **my ambitions** were pretty much associated with things that may be quantified, like book sales, and now my ambitions are mainly *"Did I do employment that helped someone get better"?*
Or" improve their health"?
" Or did I do something that actually helped me connect with someone"?
These are **the ways** I measure my success

Now she is currently within the business of writing **health books concerning;** problems associated with the kidneys, heart, diabetes, she collaborates with some **medical journals**, within the creation of recipes which will help readers who attempt to keep their pathologies

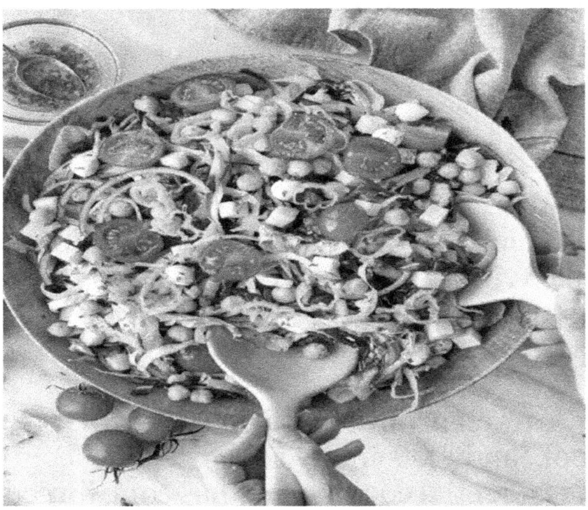

	A1 Normal to very mildly increased urine protein levels	**A2** Moderately increased urine protein levels	**A3** Severely increased urine protein levels
G1 Normal kidney function. *90% and over*	low risk of disease progression	moderately increased risk of disease progression	high risk of disease progression
G2 Mildly decreased kidney function (relative to normal range for young adult). *60-89%*	low risk of disease progression	moderately increased risk of disease progression	high risk of disease progression
G3a Mild-moderate loss of kidney function. *45-59%*	moderately increased risk of disease progression	high risk of disease progression	very high risk of disease progression
G3b Moderate-severe loss of kidney function. *30-44%*	high risk of disease progression	very high risk of disease progression	very high risk of disease progression
G4 Severe loss of kidney function. *15-29%*	very high risk of disease progression	very high risk of disease progression	very high risk of disease progression
G5 Kidney failure. *Less than 15% of function remaining*	very high risk of disease progression	very high risk of disease progression	very high risk of disease progression

- **Not considered to be Chronic Kidney Disease unless there is other evidence of kidney damage, e.g. abnormalities on scans or evidence of filter damage (glomerulonephritis)**
- **Mild Chronic Kidney Disease (due to mildly or moderately changing kidney function and urine protein levels)**
- **Chronic Kidney Disease**
- **End-Stage Kidney Disease**

Introduction

Some of the emergences of life exist into what we label "Food." We understand that food might include a range of vitamins and minerals, lots of enzymes to helped to boost digestion, dozens of phytonutrients (real organic nutrients and solvents) that retard aging and deter disease states, fiber, amino acids, natural sugars, and important fatty acid oxidation of which our bodies need to build safe cells as per our existing knowledge of nutrition. For the energy production needed by any cell, our bodies need healthy sugars through complex carbs. To create new organs and tissues, we require amino acids from stable proteins. Necessary fatty acids, which can be found in plants, grains, and nuts, are required to support the human brain and nervous systems and maintain stable immune systems that can combat disease.

We require enzymes to ensure that all of these foods are digested correctly so that our organisms get the foundations they need for proper cell development.

Good cells end in healthy tissues. Stable organs are made up of healthy tissues. Oral systems that are stable are made up of healthy cells. Good organ systems, in essence, result in healthy human beings. Everyone's life depends on an adequate diet.

Individuals with kidney failure ought to be aware of this. You didn't get rid of all the contaminants and liquids that develop up in the body according to what you consume, except with the aid of artificial kidney therapies (dialysis). You and your kidney dietitian will work together to create a meal schedule that is right for you that contains a few of your favorite foods. Your personalized meal schedule would be dependent on your age, weight, favorite meals,

dialysis appointments, and any other medical problems you may have, including diabetes, heart disease, or blood pressure. It will be customized to specific needs, although it will likely not suit all patients' needs. Nutrition, calcium, sodium, phosphate, and fluid must all be reduced in the diet of people with kidney disease. Each person has distinct requirements. You will feel healthier if you obey the meal plan prescribed by your kidney dietitian.

Chapter 1: What is Renal Diet?

Before discussing renal diet, let's consider the function of kidneys to get a clearer picture.

The kidneys tucked up at the back of the abdomen are virtualized mainstays. It is their task to process and extract waste materials from the body. Since it is completely possible to sustain with only a single kidney, several people do not consider them very significant. Getting afflicted with kidney disease used to be a catastrophe, but due to medical science improvements, new drugs, and therapies like dialysis, far more people can cope with kidney disease. When the kidneys get old or become weakened, they are put under more pressure to perform their tasks, and they can ultimately stop functioning smoothly.

Chronic kidney disease (CKD) is an illness that occurs due to some medical disorder, such as hypertension or diabetes. It's crucial to know, what is the function of kidneys in the body so that you can learn how kidney failure affects you. Your kidneys are in charge of:

- Filtration of sewage and water from the bloodstream.
- Maintaining proper mineral quantities for the body to work properly.
- Hormones have been produced that help control blood pressure, retain bone integrity, and generate the essential red blood cells.

This is what keeps you safe and makes you feel good. However, when the kidneys are under stress, they lose their capacity to perform these tasks and continue to deteriorate, signaling the beginning of a progression into chronic kidney disease. It is typically lifelong and can escalate over time. Even in the latter stages of the illness, many patients would have no effects at all. Chronic kidney disease may lead to various severe problems and, if left unchecked, irreversible kidney harm. End-stage renal failure is the name for this disorder. Such health issues include:

- Coronary heart disease
- Anemia
- An uptick in the probability of breaking a bone
- Hyperkalemia is a disorder in which potassium levels suddenly increase.
- Immune system deficiency

Diagnosing kidney failure, on the other hand, would not lead to the end of time. You can deal with the condition, with one of the most significant items you can do is eat a healthy diet to protect your kidneys. Here we will give you a short rundown of the renal diet, including what things you can and can't consume, as well as a few recipes to reassure you that you can enjoy a delicious range of nutritious meals. You don't have to give up delicious food when you have kidney failure!

The renal diet is intended to reduce the amount of phosphorus and protein you ingest, and you will even need to limit your sodium, potassium, and calcium intake. A renal diet will help minimize the number of wastes your body produces, easing the kidneys' pressure and allowing them to function more effectively. It may also aid in postponing the occurrence of kidney failure. You can first seek medical advice, particularly if you have other health issues, such as diabetes. We'll go into the adjustments you'll need to make to your diet in this segment.

1.1. Significant Diet Concerns

Your kidney diet "medication" can vary according to the kidney disease level, medication method, blood work, and if you have diabetes or elevated blood pressure. A renal diet could be daunting initially, but it is much simpler to execute than you would expect. The recommended nutrient intake outlined in this book will get you off to a great start while also providing you with delicious kidney-friendly recipes. The following macronutrients, vitamins, and minerals should be closely regulated to keep your kidneys as safe as possible, as shown by this chapter.

- Phosphorus
- Protein
- Potassium
- Sodium
- Calories
- Fats
- Vitamins/Minerals
- Carbohydrates

- Fluids

When you read this chapter, please bear in mind that the serving size determines whether a meal is medium, moderate, or heavy in a given nutrient. If you eat a big portion of raspberries instead of a half-cup portion, a low-potassium food becomes a high-potassium food.

1. ***Control the Phosphorus intake***

Phosphorus is a mineral that is found in nature. Phosphates are phosphorus as well as other mineral-containing salts that are present in our bones. Phosphorus, like calcium, aids in the development of sturdy and balanced bones. Healthy kidneys will remove additional phosphorus in the bloodstream. Phosphate or phosphorus compounds are present in nearly all foods, making it impossible to fully remove them from the diet.

Dairy products & milk, sardines, bran, dried beans, brown rice, quinoa, peas, millet, nuts and seeds, organ meat, amaranth, soda, and chocolate are rich in phosphorus.

Baking powder, filtered iced tea, baked products, waffles, cookies, pancakes and sodas, frozen and enriched foods, instant puddings, and sauces are high in phosphate additives. Calcium gets pulled off your bones because you get too much ammonia in the blood, leading to fragile bones. Phosphorus starts to build up when the kidneys fail, causing symptoms like extreme itching, muscle aches and pains, bone cancer, stiffening of the blood vessels, particularly those leading to the heart, and residues on the skin the joints. Low-phosphorus, medium-phosphorus, and high-phosphorus foods are mentioned in the table in the following section. Please discuss having your blood phosphorus level tested with your doctor. Phosphorus in the diet should be reduced to 800 to 1,000 milligrams a day for patients with chronic kidney failure and others on dialysis.

- **Limit food rich in phosphorus**

  Meats, eggs, dairy, and fish, should be avoided (you may have one serving of 7-8 ounces). Dairy products such as milk and cheese (you may have one 4 oz. serving)

- **Avoid rich phosphorus food**

white beans, purple beans, Lima beans, black-eyed peas, red beans, and garbanzo beans are rich in phosphorus. Grains that are dark, whole, or unrefined. Doughs that can be stored in the refrigerator, such as Pillsbury's Dried fruits and vegetables, Chocolate, Dark-colored sodas.

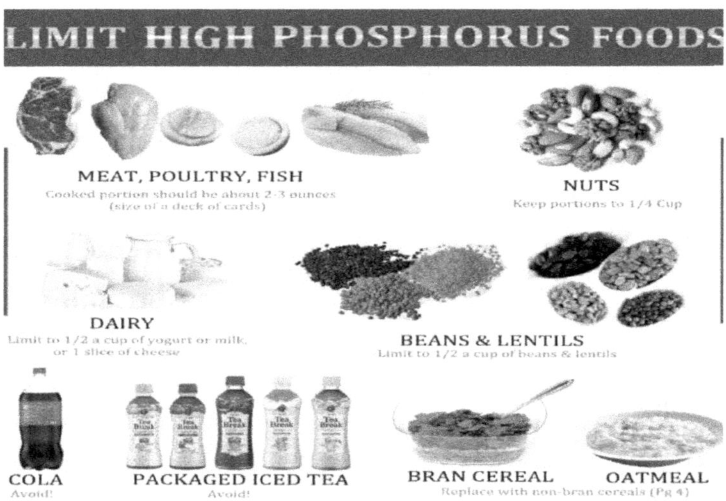

- **Remember to take phosphate binders for your meals and snacks**

A phosphate binder, a kind of polymer gel or calcium drug, may be prescribed by the doctor. You must take the phosphate binder according to your doctor's instructions. Taking a phosphate binder with each meal and snack is common. The total phosphorus consumption is typically reduced to 1000 mg.

2. *Control the protein intake*

Protein is highly essential in the human body. Protein is essential for tissue repair, muscle growth, and infection resistance. That is why protein has become so vital for maintaining health. Per day, the average human requires between 40 and 65 grams of protein. If you have chronic kidney disease in phases 1, 2, or 3, your daily protein consumption would be reduced to 12 to 15% of your total calories, which is the same amount prescribed by the Food and Nutrition board for a balanced diet on average adults. Protein intake will be limited to 10% of your daily calorie intake if you're in the fourth stage of chronic kidney disease. Protein is removed from the blood as dialysis eliminates waste. As a result, you must consume enough protein to compensate for the protein you've missed. Otherwise, the body will need to obtain protein through the muscles to meet its protein requirements. It will cause you to lose weight, become very weak, and put you at risk for infection. Dialysis patients can consume around 1.2 grams of protein per kilogram of body weight per day.

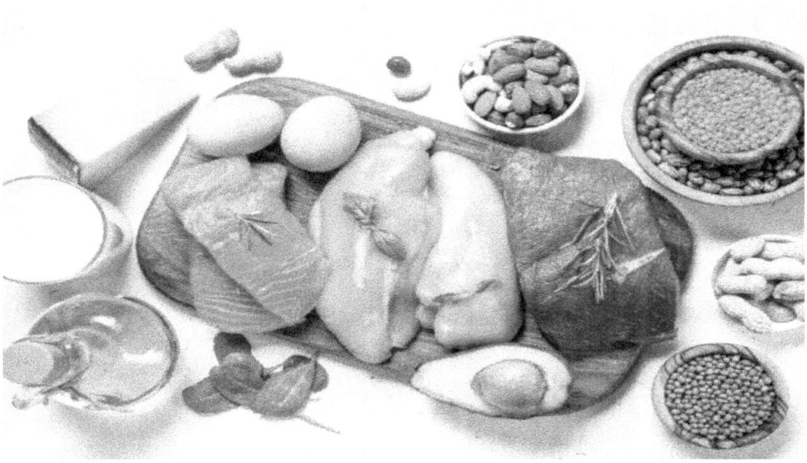

To put it another way, if you weighed 150 pounds, you'd need about 82 grams of protein a day. High-quality protein sources should account for at least half of your daily protein intake. Keeping track of how much protein you consume will prolong the life of your kidneys. Protein also aids in the battle against bacteria and the healing of wounds and provides nutrition to the body. The following are examples of products that are rich in protein and need to use in the diet.

- Eggs
- Almonds

- Pistachios
- cashews
- Chicken breast
- Cottage cheese
- Lean beef
- Parmesan cheese
- Tuna
- Swiss cheese
- Mozzarella
- Oats
- cheddar
- Greek yogurt
- Broccoli
- Milk serum protein additions
- Pulses
- Soybeans

- kidney beans
- chickpeas
- Shrimp
- Milk
- Pumpkin seeds
- Flax seeds
- sunflower seeds
- White Bread
- chia seeds
- Breast piece of Turkey
- Quinoa
- Brussels sprouts
- All kind of fish
- Peanuts

3. *Control the Potassium intake*

Potassium is an essential mineral that the body requires to maintain the heart safe and efficient. It's also important to maintain a healthy water balance amongst your cells and body fluids. Healthy kidneys excrete overabundance potassium via urination. Since the kidneys cannot expel potassium from the bloodstream when they are not operating correctly, it piles up in the body. Potassium levels in the blood that are too high or too low may be dangerous to the body. Any patients with renal disorder require more potassium than others. Potassium requirements depend greatly on how well the kidneys perform.

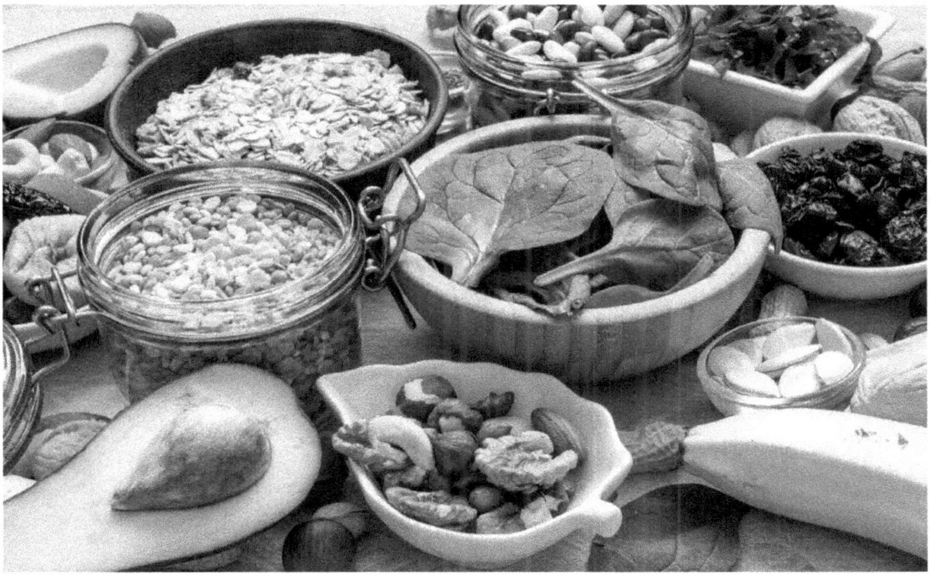

Potassium is used in all foods; however, some foods have a high potassium content. A table listing low-potassium, medium-potassium, and high-potassium foods can be found in the following section. If the blood potassium content is high, the potassium you ingest is typically not limited if you have kidney disease. Please discuss getting your blood potassium level tested with your doctor. Potassium consumption can be maintained between 2,000 and 3,000 milligrams a day while you are on dialysis.

- **High Potassium Food**
- One medium banana
- ½ of papaya
- ½ cup of prune juice
- ¼ cup of raisins
- One medium mango or kiwi
- One small orange or ½ cup of orange juice
- ½ cup of cubed cantaloupe (215) or diced honeydew melon
- One medium pear
- One medium baked potato, with skin
- One baked medium sweet potato, with skin
- ½ cup of tomato or vegetable juice or one medium raw tomato
- ½ cup of mushrooms
- ½ cup of fresh brussels sprouts

- ½ cup of cooked zucchini or winter squash
- ¼ of a medium avocado
- ½ cup of broccoli
- ½ cup of cooked pinto beans or lentils
- 1 cup of soy milk
- 3 ounces of baked or broiled salmon
- 3 ounces of roasted turkey, dark meat
- ¼ cup of sunflower seeds
- 3 ounces of cooked lean beef
- Two tablespoons of smooth peanut butter
- 6 ounces of yogurt
- 1 cup of nonfat, low-fat, or whole milk
- One slice of white bread
- ½ cup of white or brown rice
- ½ cup of spaghetti or macaroni
- One flour or corn tortilla

- One four-inch waffle
- **Medium Potassium food**
- ½ cup of ricotta cheese
- ½ cup of vanilla ice cream
- ½ cup of low-fat (2%) cottage cheese
- 1 ounce of salted peanuts, almonds, or cashews
- One large egg
- ½ cup of corn
- ½ cup of fresh or cooked carrots
- ½ cup of fresh cauliflower
- ½ cup of asparagus
- ½ cup of canned peas
- 1 cup of lettuce, all types
- ½ cup of fresh green beans
- ½ cup of frozen green beans
- ½ cup of cucumber

- One medium peach
- One small apple or ½ cup of apple juice
- ½ cup of peaches canned in juice
- ½ cup of canned pineapple
- ½ cup of fresh, sliced strawberries
- ½ cup of watermelon
- **Low potassium food**
- ½ cup of cranberries (45) or cranberry juice cocktail
- ½ cup of nectar of papaya, mango, or pear
- 1 ounce of cheese

4. Control the sodium intake

Sodium is a component that aids in the regulation of water level and blood pressure in the body. When your kidneys are healthy, they can extract sodium from the bloodstream if required, so when they aren't, sodium can pile up in the body, causing high blood pressure, fluid retention, and dehydration. Your kidney failure is more likely to worsen if you have high blood pressure. If you have elevated blood pressure or are accumulating liquid and are in the initial stages of progressive kidney disease (levels 1–4), you will have to undergo certain lifestyle changes. Whether you have stage 5 progressive kidney disease and require dialysis, you must eat a low-sodium diet and drink not increases than 1,500 mg of sodium each day or around a teaspoon of salt. (It's interesting to remember that the highest amount of sodium you're given every day is one teaspoon, which covers all foods plus extra salt.) To keep the blood pressure under control, stick to a sodium-restricted diet. Managing your blood pressure will help you avoid heart failure & slow the progression of renal disease.

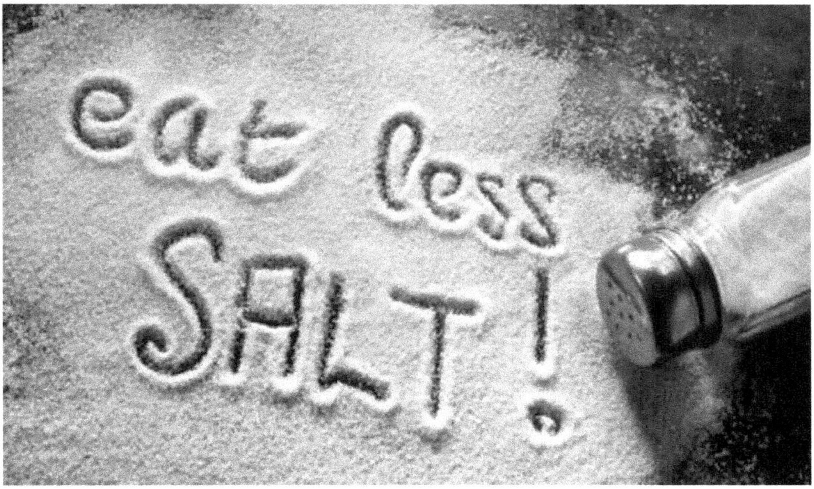

- **High sodium meals**
- Salted, cured, smoked, & canned meat, poultry or fish, cold cuts, bacon, ham, caviar, frankfurters, sardines, anchovies, and sausages.
- Frosty meats & dinners, like Pizza & burritos.
- Tinned appetizers, like spam, ravioli, also chili.
- Salty nuts, beans packed with added salt, Buttermilk.

- Natural and treated cheese, sauces, Cottage cheese & cheese spreads.
- Rolls and slices of bread with brackish tops.
- Self-ascending flour, pancakes, biscuit, Quickbread, waffle mixes, Pizza, breadstick or croutons, and salty crackers.
- Prepacked treated mixes for pasta, potatoes, rice, or fillings.
- Regular tinned vegetables and veggie juices.
- Sauerkraut, pickles, Olives, and other pickled vegetables.
- Veggies prepared with salted pork, bacon, & ham.
- Packed mixes, like crenated & Au gratin potatoes, Tater Tots & freezing hash browns.
- Store-bought readymade pasta, salsa, or tomato sauces.
- Regular canned and dehydrated soup, broth, bouillon Cup of noodles and seasoned ramen

mixes, seasoning salt, Soy sauce, additional sauces, and marinades.

- Prepacked salad dressings, normal salad dressing with cured ham bits, Saline butter or margarine, cake, Instant pudding, Hefty servings of ketchup, and mustard.
- **Low sodium food**
- Any kind of fresh or preserved fish, beef, pork, lamb, poultry.
- Eggs and also egg substitutes, reduced-sodium peanut butter.
- Dry peas & beans (not tinned)
- Tinned fish Drained, aquatic or oil-packed preserved fish or hens.
- Yogurt, ice creams, milk, and slush milk.
- Reduced sodium ricotta cheese, mozzarella cheese, and cream cheese.
- Bagels, bread also rolls without salty tops. Pancakes and utmost readymade cereals.

- All pasta & rice, nonetheless add salt while boiling.
- Reduced sodium corn, flour tortillas, also noodles.
- Reduced-sodium crackers or bread-sticks.
- Unsalted pretzels, popcorn, and chips.
- Fresh and icy vegetables are deprived of sauces.
- Low-sodium canned vegetables, sauces, and juices.
- New potatoes, ice-covered French fries, and readymade mashed potatoes.
- Reduced-salt tomatoes & V-8 juices.
- Utmost fresh, cold, and preserved fruit and dehydrated fruits.
- Reduced-sodium tinned and dried broths, soup also bouillon.
- Homebased broths deprived of added salt, unsalted butter, vinegar, margarine, Vegetable oils.

- Reduced sodium salsa, sauces, mayonnaise, and salad dressings.
- All desserts are prepared, deprived of salt.

5. *Control the calories intake*

Calories are found in all things we consume that provide us with the energy we need to survive daily. While you suffer from kidney disease, particularly if you are on dialysis, the calorie requirements are higher. Since you have stage 3 or 4 chronic kidney disease, your doctor can recommend dietary changes, particularly if you are not at a good weight. Depending on the situation, you might be advised to lose or gain a few pounds. Maintaining a good weight will help manage kidney disease and the prevention of further health issues. A balanced weight-loss program normally improves blood pressure and blood sugar levels. As a result, further kidney damage can be delayed or avoided. Whenever you need to increase your calorie intake to increase weight, the easiest way to do so is to have one high-fat item in each meal or snack. The normal calorie requirements for chronic kidney disease and dialysis are 30 to 35 calories per kilogram of body weight. While you weigh 150 pounds, this equates to about 2,000 calories a day.

6. *Control the fat intake*

You will need to minimize the level of fat you consume while your blood lipid (fat) rates are elevated. There is a connection between renal disease and cardiovascular disease. Kidney disease and other complications, including diabetes and elevated blood pressure, are implicated as the cause of heart disease. It is preferable to consume healthier fats such as olive oil or canola oil. Almonds, avocados, and seeds may be used in your diet if your blood phosphorus and potassium are limited enough. Tuna and salmon are both high in heart-healthy fats, making them a nutritious option for the diet. The key is to limit your fat consumption by about less than 30% of your daily calorie intake. If your daily calorie intake is 2,000 calories, the fat calories should be reduced to 600 calories (roughly 70 grams).

7. *Control vitamins & minerals supplements*

Over-the-counter multivitamins may be detrimental to your health whether you have renal disease or are on dialysis. Since doses of vitamins K, E, and A stack up the body when kidney function declines, they must be reduced or even eliminated. Some multivitamins, like folic acid and B-complex, are deficient in water-soluble vitamins. Since these vitamins cannot accumulate in the body and must be supplemented regularly, you will need more of them. Have an appointment with the doctor to get a recommendation for a kidney multivitamin.

8. *Carbohydrates or fiber*

Fiber is used in certain carbohydrate-containing foods and plays a significant role in shielding the heart, circulatory system, and intestine. A rich-fiber diet can lead to weight loss and lower cholesterol, lowering your risk of cardiovascular disease. Indigestion and diarrhea are common symptoms of kidney disease. Fiber will assist you in regulating the weight and blood glucose levels while still reducing these effects. For patients with chronic kidney disorders on dialysis, at least 25 grams of fiber a day are required.

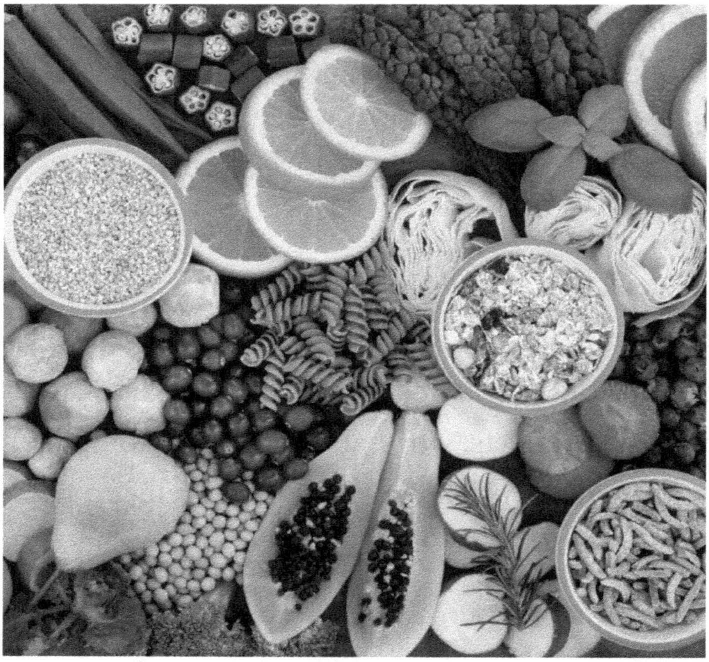

Due to calcium, phosphate, and fluid limits, this is difficult to do on a renal diet. Don't stress over consuming a minimum number of grams of fiber. While remaining under the fluid cap, try to include more high-fiber foods, which are also kidney diet-friendly. Below is a sample of foods that are rich in fiber.

- Beans
- Nuts

- Broccoli
- Berries
- Popcorn
- Whole Grains
- Apples
- Avocados
- Dried Fruits
- Potatoes

9. *Control the fluid intake*

You might need to restrict your fluid intake based on the level of kidney disease. Every food or beverage that becomes liquid at room temperature is referred to as fluid., curry, tea, milk goods, chocolate, ice cream juice, Ice milk, soups, soft drinks, sauces, jelly ice chips, and gelatin, custard, and yogurt are also included.

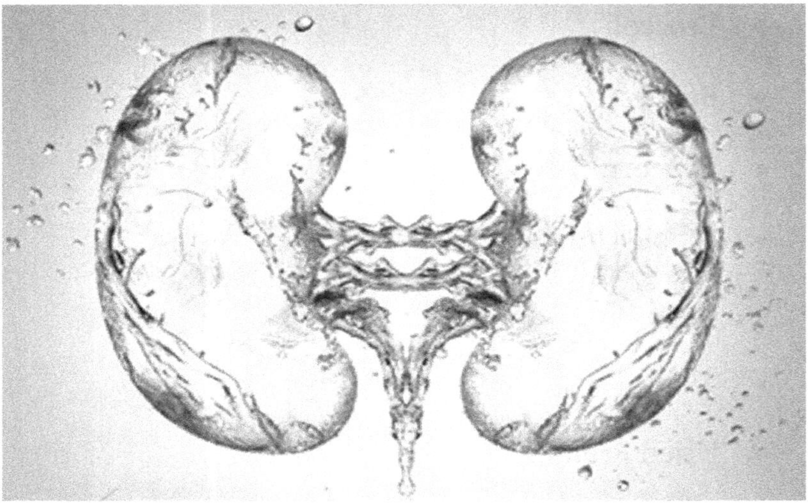

Fluid retention can occur if you drink enough water, which can cause high blood pressure and swelling, and heart failure. It would help if you drank a regular volume of fluid in the initial stages of progressive kidney disease. Your recommended fluid consumption will be determined by your urinary production, liquid buildup, and blood pressure as you progress and undergo dialysis. When you're on dialysis, your liquid intake is normally restricted to 32 to 48 ounces (1,000 to 1,500 ml.) a day.

Some information's about CDK

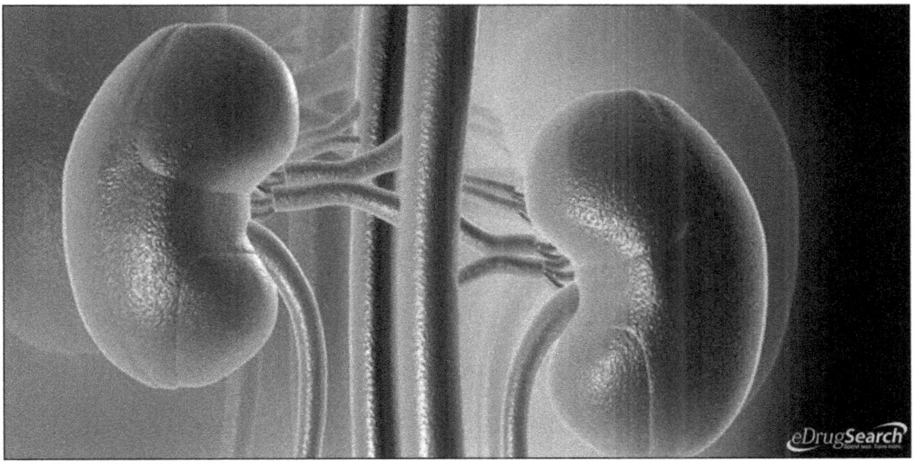

How is CKD measured and divided into stages?
Kidney disease is measured and categorised employing a biopsy which gauges the eGFR (estimated glomerular filtration rate) and a urine test which shows the ACR (urine albumin:creatinine ratio).

Glomerular filtration rate: GFR and eGFR
The main function of the kidneys is to clear water-soluble waste products (such as creatinine) from the blood. The efficiency of clearance is measured using the GFR

The GFR (glomerular filtration rate) could be a measure of what proportion blood (in millilitres) is 'cleaned' by the kidneys in one minute. By employing a biopsy to live creatinine levels we will calculate the estimated GFR, referred to as eGFR. We do that employing a formula that takes body size into consideration. the typical figure size is 1.73 m2. a traditional GFR is around 100 ml/min/1.73m2.

Because the common normal eGFR is 100, the eGFR is seen as a percentage of normal kidney function. However, values as low as 60 are considered normal if there's no other evidence of uropathy.

The eGFR is employed to calculate the 'G stage' of CKD (as indicated within the Stages of CKD chart)

The eGFR calculation are often inaccurate in those that have far more, or much less muscle than average people of their age, sex, and ethnic origin. for example, it will be falsely low in body builders, and falsely high in people with anorexia.

Albuminuria: the urine albumin: creatinine ratio

A simple urine test called the urine Albumin: Creatinine ratio (ACR) is additionally performed to appear for signs that protein is leaking into the urine (a condition called albuminuria or proteinuria). this is often a vital sign of kidney damage. The ACR is employed to calculate the 'A stage' of CKD (as indicated within the Stages of CKD chart below).

There are three recognised stages of albuminuria:

A1 – normal to mildly increased urine protein levels (lower than 3mg/mmol)

A2 – moderately increased urine protein levels (between 3-30mg/mmol)

A3 – severely increased urine protein levels (higher than 30mg/mmol)

Combining your ACR ratio along with your eGFR can help doctors attempt to predict whether your uropathy is probably going to progress and whether you're more likely to develop complications like heart and circulatory problems. Other factors are taken into consideration, e.g. age. In general, the upper the 'A' stage, the more likely it's that you just will have the benefit of blood pressure-lowering treatment.

	A1 Normal to very mildly increased urine protein levels	A2 Moderately increased urine protein levels	A3 Severely increased urine protein levels
G1 Normal kidney function. *90% and over*	**low risk of disease progression**	**moderately increased risk of disease progression**	**high risk of disease progression**
G2 Mildly decreased kidney function (relative to normal range for young adult). *60-89%*	**low risk of disease progression**	**moderately increased risk of disease progression**	**high risk of disease progression**
G3a Mild-moderate loss of kidney function. *45-59%*	**moderately increased risk of disease progression**	**high risk of disease progression**	**very high risk of disease progression**
G3b Moderate-severe loss of kidney function. *30-44%*	**high risk of disease progression**	**very high risk of disease progression**	**very high risk of disease progression**
G4 Severe loss of kidney function. *15-29%*	**very high risk of disease progression**	**very high risk of disease progression**	**very high risk of disease progression**
G5 Kidney failure. *Less than 15% of function remaining*	**very high risk of disease progression**	**very high risk of disease progression**	**very high risk of disease progression**

Not considered to be Chronic Kidney Disease unless there is other evidence of kidney damage, e.g. abnormalities on scans or evidence of filter damage (glomerulonephritis)

Mild Chronic Kidney Disease (due to mildly or moderately changing kidney function and urine protein levels)

Chronic Kidney Disease

End-Stage Kidney Disease

Remember...

Eating Right for Chronic Kidney Disease

You may have to change what you eat to manage your chronic Kidney Didease (CKD). Work with a registered dietitian to develop a hotel plan that has foods that you just enjoy eating while maintaining your kidney health.

The steps below will facilitate your eat right as you manage your CKD. the primary three steps (1-3) are important for all people with uropathy. The last two steps (4-5) may become important as your kidney function goes down.

The first steps to eating right

Step 1: Choose and prepare foods with less salt and sodium

Why? to assist control your blood pressure. Your diet should contain but 2,300 milligrams of sodium on a daily basis.

• Buy food often. Sodium (a part of salt) is added to several prepared or packaged foods you get at the supermarket or at restaurants.

• Cook foods from scratch rather than eating prepared foods, "fast" foods, frozen dinners, and canned foods that are higher in sodium. once you prepare your own food, you control what goes into it.

• Use spices, herbs, and sodium-free seasonings in situ of salt.

• Check for sodium on the Nutrition Facts label of food packages. A Daily Value of 20 percent or more means the food is high in sodium.

• Try lower-sodium versions of frozen dinners and other convenience foods.

• Rinse canned vegetables, beans, meats, and fish with water before eating.

Look for food labels with words like sodium free or salt free; or low, reduced, or no salt or sodium; or unsalted or lightly salted.

Nutrition Facts

Serving Size 1/4 Cup (30g)
Servings Per Container About 38

Amount Per Serving	
Calories 200 Calories from Fat 150	
	% Daily Value*
Total Fat 17g	**26%**
Saturated Fat 2.5g	**13%**
Trans Fat 0g	
Cholesterol 0mg	**0%**
Sodium 120mg	**5%**
Total Carbohydrate 7g	**2%**
Dietary Fiber 2g	**8%**
Sugars 1g	
Protein 5g	
Vitamin A 0% • Vitamin C 0%	
Calcium 4% • Iron 8%	

*Percent Daily Values are based on a 2,000 calorie diet.

explore for sodium on the food label. A food label showing a Percent Daily Value of fifty or less is low sodium. Also rummage around for the number of saturated and trans fats listed on the label.

Step 2: Eat the correct amount and therefore the right styles of protein

Why? to assist protect your kidneys. When your body uses protein, it produces waste. Your kidneys remove this waste. Eating more protein than you would like may make your kidneys work harder.

- Eat small portions of protein foods.
- Protein is found in foods from plants and animals. the general public eat both sorts

of protein. sit down with your dietitian about a way to choose the proper combination of protein foods for you.

Animal-protein foods:

- Chicken
- Fish
- Meat
- Eggs
- Dairy

A cooked portion of chicken, fish, or meat is about 2 to three ounces or about the scale of a deck of cards. a little of dairy foods is ½ cup of milk or yogurt, or one slice of cheese.

Plant-protein foods:

- Beans
- Nuts
- Grains

A portion of cooked beans is about ½ cup, and some of nuts is ¼ cup. a little of bread may be a single slice, and a little of cooked rice or cooked noodles is ½ cup.

Step 3: Choose foods that are healthy for your heart

Why? to assist keep fat from increase in your blood vessels, heart, and kidneys.

• Grill, broil, bake, roast, or stir-fry foods, rather than deep frying.

• Cook with nonstick cooking spray or a little amount of vegetable oil rather than butter.

• Trim fat from meat and take away skin from poultry before eating.

• Try to limit saturated and trans fats. Read the food label.

Heart-healthy foods:

• Lean cuts of meat, like loin or round

• Poultry without the skin

• Fish

- Beans
- Vegetables
- Fruits
- Low-fat or fat-free milk, yogurt, and cheese

Learn more about heart-healthy eating NIH .
Choose heart-healthy foods to assist protect your blood vessels, heart, and kidneys.

Limit alcohol

Drink alcohol only in moderation: no quite one drink per day if you're a girl, and no over two if you're a person. Drinking an excessive amount of alcohol can damage the liver, heart, and brain and cause serious health problems. Ask your health care provider what proportion alcohol you'll be able to drink safely.

The next steps to eating right

As your kidney function goes down, you will must eat foods with less phosphorus and potassium. Your health care provider will use lab tests to test phosphorus and potassium levels in your blood, and you'll be able to work along with your dietitian to regulate your design. More information is provided within the NIDDK health topic, **Nutrition for Advanced Chronic Kidney Disease.**

Step 4:Choose foods and drinks with less

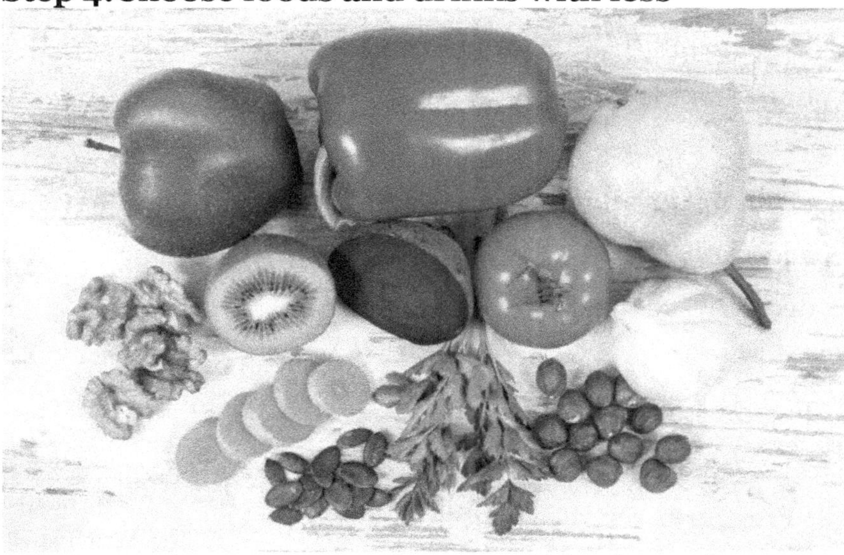

Why? to assist protect your bones and blood vessels. once you have CKD, phosphorus can build up in your blood. an excessive amount of phosphorus in your blood pulls calcium from your bones, making your bones thin, weak, and more likely to interrupt. High levels of phosphorus in your blood can even cause itchy skin, and bone and joint pain.

• Many packaged foods have added phosphorus. explore for phosphorus—or for words with “PHOS”—on ingredient labels.

• Deli meats and a few fresh meat and poultry can have added phosphorus. Ask the butcher to assist you decide fresh meats without added phosphorus.

Foods Lower in Phosphorus

• Fresh fruits and vegetables
• Breads, pasta, rice
• Rice milk (not enriched)
• Corn and rice cereals
• Light-colored sodas/pop, like lemon-lime or homemade iced tea

Foods Higher in Phosphorus

- Meat, poultry, fish
- Bran cereals and oatmeal
- Dairy foods
- Beans, lentils, nuts
- Dark-colored sodas/pop, punch, some bottled or canned iced teas that have added phosphorus

Your health care provider may check with you about taking a phosphate binder with meals to lower the quantity of phosphorus in your blood. A phosphate binder may be a medicine that acts sort of a sponge to absorb, or bind, phosphorus while it's within the stomach. Because it's bound, the phosphorus doesn't get into your blood. Instead, your body removes the phosphorus through your stool.

Step 5: Choose foods with the proper amount of potassium

Why? to assist your nerves and muscles work the correct way. Problems can occur when blood potassium levels are too high or too low. Damaged kidneys allow potassium to make up in your blood, which might cause serious heart problems.

Your food and drink choices can facilitate your lower your potassium level, if needed.

- Salt substitutes is very high in potassium.

 Read the ingredient label. seek advice from your provider about using salt substitutes.

- Drain canned fruits and vegetables before eating.

Foods Lower in Potassium

- Apples, peaches
- Carrots, green beans
- White bread and pasta
- White rice
- Rice milk (not enriched)
- Cooked rice and wheat cereals, grits
- Apple, grape, or cranberry juice

Foods Higher in Potassium

- Oranges, bananas, and fruit juice
- Potatoes, tomatoes
- Brown and wild rice
- Bran cereals
- Dairy foods
- Whole-wheat bread and pasta
- Beans and nuts

Some medicines can also raise your potassium level. Your health care provider may adjust the medicines you are taking.

View tips for people with chronic kidney disease:

- **Sodium (PDF, 167.43 KB)**
- **Phosphorus (PDF, 529.67 KB)**
- **Potassium (PDF, 158.93 KB)**
- **Protein (PDF, 1.15 MB)**

Physical Activity in Patients with Chronic Kidney Disease:

Exercise and physical activity of any kind provide a considerable number of health benefits. In fact, the 2018 Physical Activity Guidelines from the American College of medicine (ACSM) recommend that some exercise is healthier than none.

However, 150 minutes of moderate-intensity exercise per week remains the 'gold-standard' for adults to achieve substantial health benefits.

Physical activity can make people feel, function, and sleep better, and reduce the chance of an outsized number of chronic diseases.

The evidence about the health benefits gained from regular physical activity is well established, however, we still conduct research to grasp what works to induce people moving and to supply insight on how exercise can benefit various patient populations.

The 2018 ACSM Physical Activity Guidelines expanded on the physical activity recommendations for adults living with chronic conditions. These recommendations developed as we've got gained a stronger understanding that certain modalities and intensity of exercise don't seem to be necessarily the simplest options for everybody.

There are variety of chronic conditions and disabilities, but the ACSM Guidelines particularly focused on activity in adults living with osteoarthritis, **type 2 diabetes**, hypertension, adult cancer survivors, **Parkinson's disease**, degenerative disorder, medulla spinalis injury, and stroke. supported current guidelines, those living with a chronic condition or disability, if able, should do:

- **At least 150 to 300 minutes** every week of moderate-intensity, or 75 to 150 minutes of vigorous-intensity aerobic physical activity.

- **Muscle-strengthening activities** of moderate or greater intensity that involve all major muscle groups on 2 or more days per week.

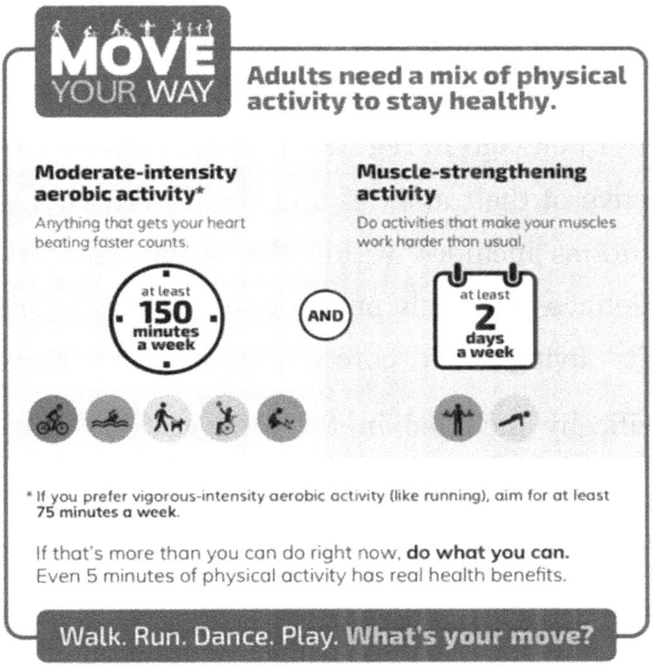
MOVE
YOUR WAY
Adults need a mix of physical activity to stay healthy.
Moderate-intensity aerobic activity*
Anything that gets your heart beating faster counts.
at least
150
minutes
a week
AND
Muscle-strengthening activity
Do activities that make your muscles work harder than usual.
at least
2
days
a week
* If you prefer vigorous-intensity aerobic activity (like running), aim for at least 75 minutes a week.
If that's more than you can do right now, do what you can.
Even 5 minutes of physical activity has real health benefits.
Walk. Run. Dance. Play. What's your move?

Research has demonstrated that the mixture of aerobic and strength training can provide additional health benefits, particularly to those living with chronic conditions. Perhaps most significant, the rules emphasize that if adults living with chronic conditions or disabilities are unable to satisfy the above recommendations, they ought **to engage in regular physical activity t**o the most effective of their abilities and avoid inactivity. While the conditions included within the ACSM Physical Activity Guidelines are highly prevalent conditions within the us, adults living with chronic nephrosis (CKD) weren't specifically included in these suggestions· Exercise has many known benefits, and also the current evidence supports the concept that regular physical activity in specific patient populations can have greater health benefits for these individuals. It is estimated that 30 million adults within the u. s. have some stage of CKD, one in every of the foremost costly diseases within the world. Therapies to enhance outcomes and slow disease progression remain inadequate.

Physical dysfunction and muscle atrophy are often observed in patients with CKD and both contribute to a loss of independence and functional status- two important priorities to patients with CKD. More importantly, the progression of inactivity and muscle atrophy appear to extend with the worsening of CKD overtime. Given a number of the limited physical function of patients with CKD, there's great potential that tiny amounts of exercise could have meaningful, positive impacts on their wellbeing.

More importantly, could exercise help slow the progression of CKD? In a review by Drs. Johansen and Painter, they discuss the association between physical activity and kidney function, however this relationship remains controversial.

A study from 2008 had patients with CKD (mean estimated glomerular filtration rate [eGFR] 29.9±17.0 mL/min/1.73 m2) complete a stress test (peak oxygen uptake), physical performance measures (sit to face, gait speed, and 6-minute walk), and health status questionnaires.

The authors failed to observe a correlation between maximal oxygen consumption (VO2peak) and eGFR, but a correlation between maximal gait speed and eGFR was observed. In contrast to the present study, Clyne et al observed a major positive relationship between GFR and maximal exercise capacity after adjustment for age, sex, and hemoglobin concentration in men and ladies with CKD (GFR starting from 3-32 mL/min/1.73 m2). In human studies, there appears to be an overall positive relationship between exercise and slowing CKD progression, with exercise improving various markers of kidney function decline. However, the disagreement between the results of those studies may be associated with the heterogeneity of CKD, the modality and intensity of exercise used, the result measures, and poor study design (not controlling for sex, age, stage of disease, baseline values, etc).

The heterogeneity of nephrosis in humans may be a confounding factor we can't control for, however, the utilization of animal models provides a chance to raised understand how exercise can more directly impact CKD progression.

Avin et al is an example of a study that took advantage of utilizing an animal model to further investigate the impact of exercise in nephrosis. during this study, researchers utilized a rat model of progressive polycystic CKD (Cy/+IU on a Hans-Sprague Daley background) to research the hypothesis that voluntary wheel running would improve musculoskeletal health and slow uropathy progression.

This rodent model features a mutation in **Anks6**, encoding for the protein SamCystin located at the bottom of cilia, and alters the nephronophthisis complex.

Rats with this mutation spontaneously develop CKD with mineral-bone disorder that corresponds to stage 2-3 CKD in humans. during this study, researchers decided to model human access to exercise by providing a freely accessible activity wheel for the rodents to voluntarily utilize over the course of the study.

- At 25 weeks old, male rats got access to a voluntary running wheel or a typical cage condition (no wheel) for 10 weeks.
- Cage activity, grip strength, maximal aerobic capacity, and body composition were measured at both the beginning and end of the study.
- At the top of the ten weeks, serum biochemistries (creatinine, phosphorus, parathyroid hormone), tissue weight, and bone micro-CT and mechanics were measured.
- The key findings from this study were:
- Male rats with uropathy ran but wild-type littermate rats.
- An inverse relationship with disease progression and physical activity was observed, meaning that as renal disorder progressed, the gap the rats ran decreased additionally
- . Exercise had some benefit in rats with renal disorder.

- Overall statistical significant improvements in serum biochemistries within the rats with nephropathy that got access to a wheel:
- creatinine: 1.26±0.9 vs 0.99±0.58 mg/dL
- phosphorus: 6.14±1.09 vs 5.17±1.31 mg/dL
- parathyroid hormone: 803±539 vs 521±198 pg/mL
- This is relevant to human patients with polycystic nephropathy that ends up in kidney functional decline and confirms that nephropathy itself is related to a progressive decline in physical activity, independent old and comorbid conditions (both controlled for within the study). These findings are in line with those from human studies, and here suggest that even some voluntary exercise had a beneficial effect on disease progression during this model.

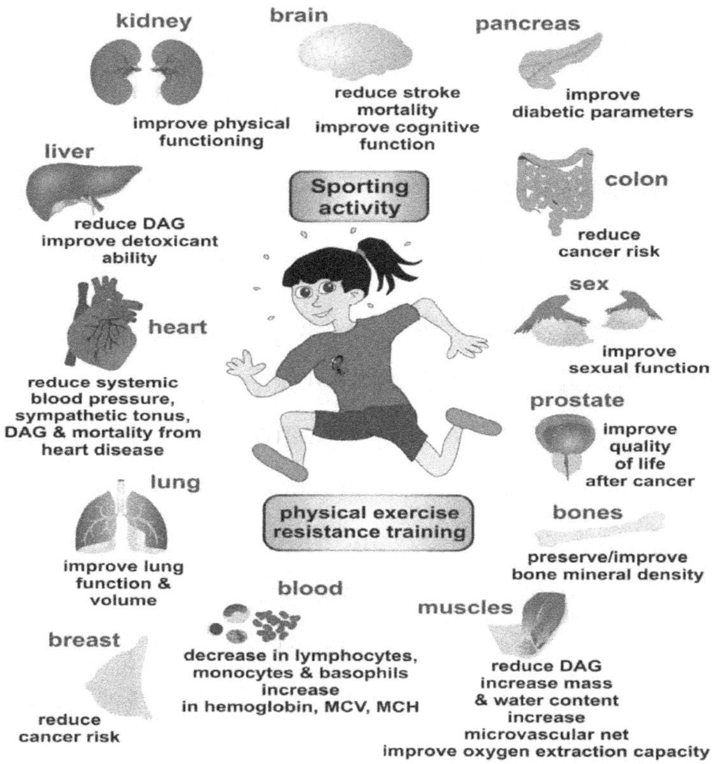
kidney
improve physical functioning
brain
reduce stroke mortality
improve cognitive function
pancreas
improve diabetic parameters
liver
reduce DAG
improve detoxicant ability
Sporting activity
colon
reduce cancer risk
heart
reduce systemic blood pressure, sympathetic tonus, DAG & mortality from heart disease
sex
improve sexual function
prostate
improve quality of life after cancer
lung
improve lung function & volume
physical exercise
resistance training
bones
preserve/improve bone mineral density
blood
decrease in lymphocytes, monocytes & basophils
increase in hemoglobin, MCV, MCH
muscles
reduce DAG
increase mass & water content
increase microvascular net
improve oxygen extraction capacity
breast
reduce cancer risk

Using a different animal model of CKD (spontaneously hypertensive rats [SHR] with a ⅚ nephrectomy), **Kohzuki** et al assessed the effect of moderate chronic treadmill exercise on kidney function. This study also included antihypertensive therapy in an exceedingly few of the groups, except for the aim of this post, we are that specialize in the exercise vs non-exercise groups only.

Male mice were subjected to exercise training employing a treadmill at 20 m/min, 0 grade incline, for hour,

- 5 days every week for 4 weeks (this intensity corresponds to 65% of VO2max). pressure level, weight,
- 24 hour urine volume, urinary Na+, K+, and urinary protein were measured before and after exercise hebdomadally. Following the 4 weeks of coaching, animals were sacrificed to work out serum protein, albumin, glucose, urea nitrogen (BUN), creatinine, total cholesterol, and triglycerides. Focal glomerular sclerosis (IGS) was also determined with the kidney remnants.

After 4 weeks of moderate

- exercise training, this study found that: Exercise has kidney-protective effects during this rodent model.
- Urinary protein excretion was significantly reduced in rodents within the exercise condition compared to non-exercise animals.
- Moderate exercise training significantly protected against increases in IGS.

Using two different models of nephrosis, Kohzuki et al and Avin et al provided support for exercise to assist slow the progression of CKD. One observation from the Avin et al study that stuck bent me specifically, was that the animals with nephrosis and access to an activity wheel were more active than those with uropathy and no wheel access, despite no incentive to be more active.

While the non-exercise group failed to have access to a wheel, and so, after all were less active, these findings suggest that simply providing access to physical activity could increase overall activity in patients with CKD.

This observation is intriguing since more often than not, the first reasons for low physical activity are access and time. Patients with CKD who receive dialysis treatments often do so **2-3 times** every week and may therefore be limited in both extra personal time and access to safe and healthy exercise options. However, this study suggests that simply providing the access for patients could increase activity levels in these individuals.

However, it's important to notice that human behavior and motivation are extremely complex, and therefore the human environment isn't as easily controlled. Nonetheless, it's possible that incorporating opportunities for physical activity in treatment plans for patients with renal disorder could improve their health and care. Current basic and clinical research present exciting observations that highlight the potential benefits of moderate intensity exercise among patients with uropathy. Importantly, the activity levels described within the basic studies discussed here align with the 2018 ACSM Physical Activity Guidelines, that any activity is healthier than no activity. For patients that are limited in time and mobility, like patients with CKD, providing access and allowing people to dictate their own intensity, may provide greater benefits than a strict regimen. While some basic and clinical studies have revealed potential benefits of exercise for patients with renal disorder, there's still a big amount of research that has to be done to higher our understanding of how exercise specifically benefits patients with CKD.

1. **https://www.ncbi.nlm.nih.gov/pmc/articles/PMC3637339/**

2. **https://www.uhb.nhs.uk/Downloads/pdf/PiDietaryAdviceKidneyFailure.pdf**

3. **https://www.nejm.org/doi/full/10.1056/NEJMra1700312**

4. **https://www.ajkd.org/article/S0272-6386(20)30726-5/fulltext**

5. **https://pubmed.ncbi.nlm.nih.gov/11846025/**

6. **https://www.nature.com/articles/s41467-020-16559-0**

7. **https://www.nature.com/articles/s41598-020-75405-x**

8. **https://www.sciencedirect.com/science/article/pii/S2013251420300742**

Chapter 2: Stews & Soups

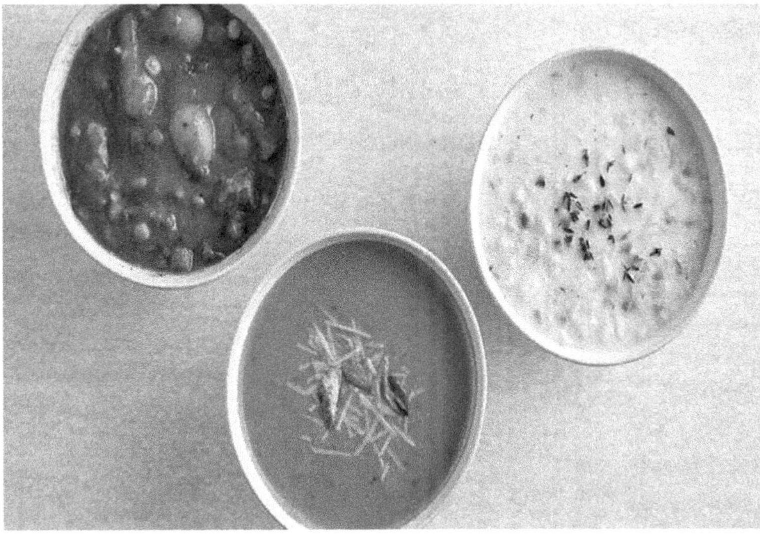

As soon as the weather starts to cool, a decent soup or stew recipe is a must-have. This collection includes some soup recipes as well as a few flavor-packed stews. Soup and stew shouldn't have to be exclusive to the fall and winter seasons, but they can certainly be a complete meal independently. This list will help you rethink how good soups could be at mealtime. You'll notice how convenient it is to prepare, how tasty it is, and also how your family would enjoy the soups or stews.

1. Soup of watercress cream

This exquisite soup's stunning pastel hue and the lush accent taste of grilled garlic make it a great recipe for hosting. You may make it for a quick family dinner, but to do the soup justice, arrange the table with china plates and solid silverware.

Time to prepare: 15 minutes

Total time: 1 hour 10 minutes

Servings: 4 persons

Ingredients

- 1 teaspoon unsalted butter
- ½ teaspoon olive oil
- ½ sweet onion, chopped
- 1 tablespoon freshly squeezed lemon
- 4 cups chopped watercress
- ¼ cup heavy cream
- ¼ cup chopped fresh parsley
- 3 cups water

- 6 garlic cloves

Instructions

1. Set the oven at 400 degrees Fahrenheit.
2. On a sheet of, aluminum foil put the garlic cloves. Glaze the foil with olive oil and roll it into a little bundle. Keep the garlic cloves in a pie dish and roast for 20 minutes, or till very tender.
3. Take off the garlic from the oven and put it on a cooling rack.
4. Melt butter in a big pan over medium heat. Cook for around 4 minutes, or when the onion is tender. Sauté for five minutes with the watercress and parsley.
5. In a mixing bowl, add the water and roast garlic pulp. Get the broth to boiling, then turn it down to low heat.
6. Cook for about 20 minutes, or once the vegetables are tender.
7. Allow cooling the soup for 5 minutes before mixing it with the heavy cream in intervals in a food processor (or using a big bowl and a hand blender).

8. Put the soup back to the pot and warm over low flame until well heated.
9. Season with salt and pepper by adding lime juice.

Nutritional Facts:

- Calories: 452 kcal
- Carbs: 50g
- Fat: 27g
- Protein: 4g
- Sodium: 0mg
- Phosphorus: 98mg
- Potassium: 91mg

2. Veggie's soup

The method for making this soup can seem strange initially; however, the outcome is delicious. Grill the vegetables first, then mix the baked vegetables with chicken broth to achieve the perfect soup thickness. To quit ingesting much more sodium and potassium, use homemade chicken broth or a properly screened commercial item in your meals.

Time to prepare: 20 minutes

Total time: 1 hour

Servings: 6 persons

Ingredients

- 1 small sweet onion, cut into quarters
- Freshly ground black pepper
- ¼ cup chopped fresh basil
- 2 cups cubed eggplant
- 2 garlic cloves, crushed
- 1 tablespoon olive oil
- 2 small red bell peppers, halved

- 1 cup Easy Chicken Stock
- Water

Instructions

1. Set the oven at 350 degrees Fahrenheit.
2. In a big oven-safe baking dish, mix the onions, red peppers, eggplant, and garlic.
3. Glaze the olive oil over the veggies.
4. Barbecue for around thirty min, or when the vegetables are lightly sauteed and tender.
5. Allow the vegetables to cool slightly before peeling the peppers.
6. Blend the vegetables with the chicken stock in portions in a blender (or in a big mixing bowl with a manual blender.
7. Shift the broth to a large bowl and add quite enough water to thin it out to the perfect consistency. Get the broth to a simmer and stir in the basil.
8. Serve with a pinch of black pepper.

Nutritional Facts:

- Calories: 50 kcal
- Carbs: 5g
- Fat: 0g
- Protein: 2g
- Sodium: 120mg
- Phosphorus: 111mg
- Potassium: 74mg

3. Turkey soup

Since chicken appears to be more readily accessible in supermarkets, turkey could be ignored. Turkey is a great, nutritious alternative for that kind of soup because it's rich in calcium, zinc, and iron while still being low in calories and fat. If at all necessary, buy the natural grass-fed turkey.

Time to prepare: 25 minutes

Total time: 45 minutes

Servings: 6 persons

Ingredients

- 2 tablespoons chopped fresh parsley
- ½ pound cooked ground turkey, 93% lean
- 4 cups water
- 1 cup Easy Chicken Stock
- 1 celery stalk, chopped
- ½ sweet onion, chopped
- 1 carrot, sliced thin
- ½ cup shredded green cabbage

- ½ cup bulgur
- 2 dried bay leaves
- Freshly ground black pepper
- 1 teaspoon chopped fresh sage
- 1 teaspoon minced garlic
- 1 teaspoon olive oil
- 1 teaspoon chopped fresh thyme
- Pinch red pepper flakes

Instructions

1. Heat the oil to a large pan over medium heat. Cook for around 5 minutes, or when the turkey is cooked completely.
2. Adding the onion and garlic. Cook for 3 minutes, or until the vegetables are softened.
3. Add the celery, chicken stock, cabbage, carrot, bulgur, and bay leaves to the water.

4. Get the broth to a boil, drop to low heat, and continue to cook for 35 minutes, or when the bulgur and veggies are soft.
5. Take the bay leaves out and add the parsley, sage, thyme, and red pepper flakes, mixing to combine.
6. Serve with a pinch of black pepper.

Nutritional Facts:

- Calories: 150 kcal
- Carbs: 10g
- Fat: 2g
- Protein: 10g
- Sodium: 100mg
- Phosphorus: 89mg
- Potassium: 111mg

4. Veggies & beef soup

When cooking, aim not to split up the ground beef, so bits add a good feel. Mix the minced beef with a couple of spoons of bread crumbs, garlic powder, or thyme, and make the mixture into little balls for an enjoyable variety. When the soup has reached a boil, add the meatballs and steam for around 30 minutes, or they'll be thoroughly cooked.

Time to prepare: 15 minutes

Total time: 55 minutes

Servings: 6 persons

Ingredients

- Freshly ground black pepper
- ½ small sweet onion, chopped
- ½ cup fresh green beans, cut into one-inch pieces
- 1 cup homemade low-sodium beef broth
- 1 teaspoon minced garlic
- ½ pound extra-lean ground beef
- 2 cups water

- ½ cup long-grain white rice, uncooked
- 1 celery stalk, chopped
- 1 teaspoon chopped fresh thyme

Instructions

1. Put the minced beef in a large pan over medium heat.
2. Fry for around 6 minutes, stirring regularly or when the beef is fully browned.
3. Remove the extra fat from the pan and put in the garlic and onions.
4. Cook for around 3 minutes, or when the veggies are tender.
5. Pour the water, beef stock, rice, potatoes, and celery into a large mixing bowl.
6. Get the broth to a boil, and drop to low heat and cook for 30 minutes once the rice is done.
7. Boil for 3 minutes with the green beans and thyme.
8. Sprinkle with pepper after taking the broth from the flame.

Nutritional Facts:

- Calories: 60 kcal
- Carbs: 10g
- Fat: 4g
- Protein: 10g
- Sodium: 200mg
- Phosphorus: 111mg
- Potassium: 74mg

5. Cabbage stew with herbs

Cabbage Stew is a low-calorie, woodsy meal that requires slight time to prepare and improves with time in the fridge. This recipe yields a nice green stew, including a light herb stock. The cabbage will tender and absorb the spices; add a hot sauce dash or a spoonful pesto for a more intense taste.

Time to prepare: 20 minutes

Total time: 1 hour

Servings: 6 persons

Ingredients

- 1 teaspoon unsalted butter
- 1 cup fresh green beans, cut into one-inch pieces
- ½ large sweet onion, chopped
- 1 teaspoon chopped fresh oregano
- 2 tablespoons freshly squeezed lemon juice
- 1 teaspoon minced garlic
- 6 cups shredded green cabbage
- 3 celery stalks, chopped with the leafy tops

- Freshly ground black pepper
- 2 tablespoons chopped fresh parsley
- 1 tablespoon chopped fresh thyme
- 1 teaspoon chopped savory
- 1 scallion, both green and white parts, chopped
- Water

Instructions

1. Melt butter in a large pan over moderate flame.
2. In molten butter, cook the garlic and onions for around 3 minutes, or when the vegetables are tender.
3. Fill the pot with enough water to cover the lettuce, celery, scallion, parsley, lime juice, thyme, savory, and oregano by around 4 inches.
4. Get the broth to a boil, and drop to low heat and cook around 25 minutes, or once the vegetables are soft.
5. Boil for 3 minutes after adding the green beans.
6. Sprinkle with pepper.

Nutritional Facts:

- Calories: 318 kcal
- Carbs: 22g
- Fat: 15g
- Protein: 20g
- Sodium: 490mg
- Phosphorus: 211mg
- Potassium: 181mg

6. Chicken stew

Stew is a soothing food that is best enjoyed throughout the wintertime, but it can also be enjoyed in all seasons. Prepare it in a crockpot on reduced flame for ten hours if you want. Fry the chicken fillets and place them in the slow cooker with the ingredients' rest (excluding the cornstarch). If the sauce has to be thickened, add the cornstarch after the stew is over.

Time to prepare: 20 minutes

Total time: 1 hour

Servings: 6 persons

Ingredients

- 1 teaspoon finely chopped fresh rosemary
- 1 tablespoon olive oil
- ½ sweet onion, chopped
- 1 tablespoon minced garlic
- 2 celery stalks, sliced
- 1 cup plus 2 tablespoons water
- 1 carrot, sliced

- 1-pound boneless, skinless chicken thighs, cut into one-inch cubes
- 2 cups Easy Chicken Stock
- 1 turnip, sliced thin
- 1 tablespoon chopped fresh thyme
- Freshly ground black pepper
- 2 teaspoons cornstarch

Instructions

1. Add the olive oil to a large pan over medium heat.
2. Cook, constantly stirring, for around 6 minutes or when the chicken is nicely browned.
3. Sauté for 3 minutes with the garlic and onions.
4. Get the stew to a boil with the chicken stock, 1 cup water, carrot, celery, and turnip.
5. Lower the heat and cook around 30 minutes, or when the chicken is thoroughly cooked and moist.
6. Boil for 3 minutes more after adding the thyme and rosemary.

7. Mix the 2 teaspoons water and cornstarch in a small cup, then pour the mixture into the stew.

8. Cook for 3 to 4 minutes, or till stew thickens, mixing to add the cornstarch paste.

9. Take out from the fire and sprinkle with freshly ground black pepper.

Nutritional Facts:

- Calories: 200 kcal
- Carbs: 20g
- Fat: 1g
- Protein: 20g
- Sodium: 290mg
- Phosphorus: 131mg
- Potassium: 111mg

Chapter 3: Salads

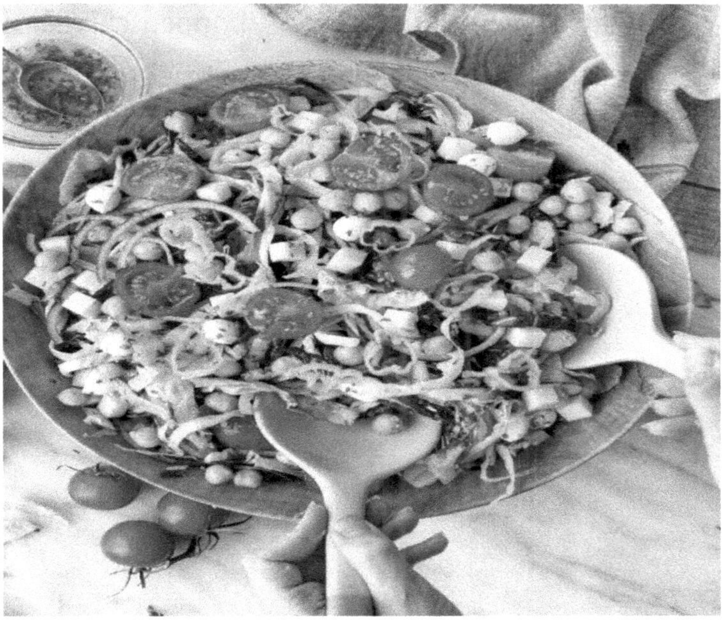

Working to be a better version of yourself? Salad recipes for healthier eating are plentiful; in general, they can be found almost everywhere.

These balanced salad ideas look so amazing that it's hard to believe they're so healthy.

Any of these dishes lift the word "salad" to new heights. Anyone trying to bring a bit more protein to the diet would love the nutritious salad recipes! Chopped salads, detox salads, green salads, chicken salads, bright fruit salads, seafood salads, and nutritious options are all accessible. Here are few recipes for delicious and unique salads.

1. Salad with strawberries & watercress with almonds topping

The almond dressing brings a surprising touch to this dish, and the nice, juicy strawberries give a burst of bright color and sweetness. Strawberries are high in vitamin C, folate, and fiber, and they are one of the top 20 fruits in terms of disease-fighting antioxidants. They will raise your positive (HDL) cholesterol and reduce blood pressure so that they may be beneficial to your heart in several ways.

Time to prepare: 15 minutes

Total time: 20 minutes

Servings: 6 persons

Ingredients

For salad dressing

- Freshly ground black pepper
- ¼ cup olive oil
- ¼ cup rice vinegar
- ¼ teaspoon pure almond extract
- 1 tablespoon honey

- ¼ teaspoon ground mustard

For salad

- 1 cup sliced strawberries
- 2 cups roughly chopped watercress
- ½ English cucumber, chopped
- 2 cups shredded green leaf lettuce
- ½ red onion, sliced very thin

Instructions

Prepare to dress

1. Mix the olive oil and rice vinegar in a medium bowl till caramelized.
2. Set aside after whisking in the honey, almond extract, mustard, and pepper.

Prepare salad

1. Mix the watercress, green lettuce, cabbage, cucumber, and strawberries in a large mixing bowl.
2. Add the salad with the dressing to mix it.

Nutritional Facts:

- Calories: 175 kcal
- Carbs: 45g
- Fat: 5g
- Protein: 4g
- Sodium: 210mg
- Phosphorus: 90mg
- Potassium: 85mg

2. Salad Waldorf

In 1893, the maître d'hôtel of the Waldorf Astoria in New York City invented the Waldorf salad. The first salad had walnuts and didn't have a sour cream sauce. This adaptation is just as delicious as the initial, and if you'd like more protein, you can top it with minced chicken.

Time to prepare: 20 minutes

Total time: 25 minutes

Servings: 4 persons

Ingredients

- 1 tablespoon granulated sugar
- 1 cup halved grapes
- 3 celery stalks, chopped
- ½ cup light sour cream
- 3 cups green leaf lettuce, torn into pieces
- 2 tablespoons freshly squeezed lemon juice
- 1 large apple, cored, peeled, and chopped

Instructions

1. Place the lettuce on four plates and set it aside.
2. Mix the grapes, celery, and apple in a shallow mixing bowl.
3. Blend the sour cream, lemon juice, and sugar in a separate small dish.
4. Toss the grape mixture with the sour cream pot. Mix to combine.
5. Divide the grape mixture evenly among the plates.

Nutritional Facts:

- Calories: 145 kcal
- Carbs: 30g
- Fat: 3g
- Protein: 2g
- Sodium: 142mg
- Phosphorus: 87mg
- Potassium: 111mg

3. Pear salad

Asian pears are the yellowish-green, oval fruit covered in a delicate slipcover and marketed alongside standard pears in the supermarket. They seem delicate, but they grate quickly without being mushy for this salad. This slaw's crisp flavor comes from these ripe, firm-textured pears. If Asian pears aren't available in your region, standard pears can be used instead.

Time to prepare: 30 minutes

Total time: 1 hour 30 minutes

Servings: 4 persons

Ingredients

- 1 cup finely shredded red cabbage
- 1 teaspoon granulated sugar
- ¼ cup olive oil
- 2 scallions, both green and white parts, chopped
- ½ cup chopped cilantro
- 2 celery stalks, chopped

- 1 Asian pear, cored and grated
- Zest of 1 lime
- 2 cups finely shredded green cabbage
- ½ red bell pepper, boiled and chopped
- Juice of 1 lime

Instructions

1. Mix the green and red cabbage with scallions, celery, pear, red pepper, and cilantro in a big mixing pot.
2. Blend the olive oil, lime juice, lime zest, and sugar in a small size bowl.
3. Put the cabbage mixture into the dressing till it is evenly distributed.
4. Before eating, chill the dish for 1 hour.

Nutritional Facts:

- Calories: 200 kcal
- Carbs: 15g
- Fat: 13g

- Protein: 3g
- Sodium: mg
- Phosphorus: 122mg
- Potassium: 104mg

4. Tabbouleh

Conventional tabbouleh is made with a substantial quantity of chopped herbs, typically mint and bulgur rather than couscous. Just a dash of olive oil and lemon juice was used in the dressing. For better results, utilize fresh juice and high-quality oil. To boost the flavors to meld, put the salad in the fridge for at minimum 1 hour.

Time to prepare: 30 minutes

Total time: 1 hour 30 minutes

Servings: 4 persons

Ingredients

- ½ red bell pepper, boiled and finely chopped
- 1 cup chopped eggplant, boiled until tender
- Zest of 1 lemon
- ¼ cup finely chopped fresh parsley
- 4 cups cooked white rice
- ¼ cup finely chopped fresh cilantro
- ½ zucchini, finely chopped, boiled until tender

- ½ yellow bell pepper, boiled and chopped
- 2 tablespoons olive oil
- Juice of 1 lemon
- Freshly ground black pepper

Instructions

1. Mix the rice, red bell pepper, yellow bell pepper, zucchini, eggplant, parsley, cilantro, olive oil, lemon juice, and lemon zest in a large mixing bowl till it's mixed.
2. Sprinkle with salt and. pepper
3. Before eating, chill the salad in the fridge for a minimum of 1 hour.

Nutritional Facts:

- Calories: 150 kcal
- Carbs: 8g
- Fat: 12g
- Protein: 4g
- Sodium: 470mg

5. Beef salad with ginger

This salad is extremely popular among people. It's easy, with fiery radishes and vibrant red onions and juicy grilled beef on top. If you want a milder taste, leave out chili paste in this recipe, as the beef marinade is already spicy. If you don't have a grill, the beef can be baked in the oven for around 6 minutes per end.

Time to prepare: 30 minutes

Total time: 1 hour 40 minutes

Servings: 6 persons

Ingredients

For beef

- 1 tablespoon grated fresh ginger
- ½ pound flank steak
- 2 tablespoons freshly squeezed lime juice
- 2 teaspoons minced garlic
- 2 tablespoons olive oil

For salad dressing

- 1 teaspoon chopped fresh thyme
- 1 tablespoon honey
- ¼ cup olive oil
- ¼ cup rice vinegar
- Zest of 1 lime
- Juice of 1 lime

For salad

- 4 cups torn green leaf lettuce
- ½ red onion, sliced thin
- ½ cup sliced radishes

Instructions

Prepare the beef

1. Mix the lemon juice, ginger, garlic, and olive oil in a medium bowl until well combined.
2. Pour the marinade over the flank steak and roll it to cover both sides.

3. Plastic wraps the bowl and marinate for one hour in the fridge.
4. Take the steak out from the marinade.
5. Set the grill temperature to moderate and cook the steak for around 5 minutes per end, rotating once, based on the steak's size.
6. Please take out the steak from the pan and put it on a chopping board to settle for ten minutes.
7. Using a sharp knife, thinly slice the beef.

Prepare vinaigrette

1. Put aside the olive oil, rice vinegar, lemon zest, lemon juice, honey, and thyme in a shallow mixing dish.

Set the salad plate

1. Divide the lettuce, onions, and radishes equally among six plates.
2. Pour vinaigrette over each salad.
3. Serve the slice of beef on top of each salad.

Nutritional Facts:

- Calories: 230 kcal
- Carbs: 11g
- Fat: 15g
- Protein: 15g
- Sodium: 660mg
- Phosphorus: 211mg
- Potassium: 163mg

6. Salad of farfalle

Whether you're off to a picnic or a BBQ, prepare this bright dish ahead of time and bring it with you. The light-colored pasta and creamy topping contrast well with the yellow, red, orange, and green vegetable tiny bits. If you want an impressive appearance, garnish with freshly diced chives and a tablespoon of lime zest.

Time to prepare: 30 minutes

Total time: 1 hour 30 minutes

Servings: 6 persons

Ingredients

- ½ teaspoon granulated sugar
- 2 cups cooked farfalle pasta
- 2 tablespoons yellow bell pepper
- Freshly ground black pepper
- ¼ cup finely chopped cucumber
- ½ scallion, green part only, finely chopped
- ¼ cup grated carrot

- ½ cup homemade mayonnaise
- 1 tablespoon freshly squeezed lemon juice
- 1 teaspoon chopped fresh parsley
- ¼ cup boiled and finely chopped red bell pepper

Instructions

1. Mix the pasta, red pepper, cucumber, carrot, yellow pepper, and scallion in a big mixing dish.
2. Blend the mayo, lime juice, parsley, and sugar in a shallow pot.
3. Mix the pasta mixture with the dressing and combine to blend.
4. Sprinkle with salt and pepper.
5. Before serving, chill for a maximum of one hour in the fridge.

Nutritional Facts:

- Calories: 170 kcal
- Carbs: 24g

- Fat: 5g
- Protein: 7g
- Sodium: 200mg
- Phosphorus: 103mg
- Potassium: 98mg

CPSIA information can be obtained
at www.ICGtesting.com
Printed in the USA
LVHW080534061021
699649LV00002B/148

9 781803 031491